MW00761595

PocketBrain of
50 UNUSUAL SYMPTOMS

POCKETBRAIN OF
50 UNUSUAL SYMPTOMS

Mark A. Marinella, MD, FACP

Assistant Clinical Professor of Medicine
Wright State University School of
Medicine
Dayton, Ohio

Practicing Hospitalist
Miami Valley Hospital
Dayton, Ohio

Blackwell
Publishing

© 2002 by Blackwell Science, Inc.
a Blackwell Publishing Company

Editorial Offices:
Commerce Place, 350 Main Street, Malden, Massachusetts 02148, USA
Osney Mead, Oxford OX2 0EL, England
25 John Street, London WC1N 2BS, England
23 Ainslie Place, Edinburgh EH3 6AJ, Scotland
54 University Street, Carlton, Victoria 3053, Australia

Other Editorial Offices:
Blackwell Wissenschafts-Verlag GmbH, Kurfürstendamm 57, 10707 Berlin, Germany
Blackwell Science KK, MG Kodenmacho Building, 7-10 Kodenmacho Nihombashi,
   Chuo-ku, Tokyo 104, Japan
Iowa State University Press, A Blackwell Science Company, 2121 S. State Avenue,
   Ames, Iowa 50014-8300, USA

Distributors:
The Americas
   Blackwell Publishing
   c/o AIDC
   P.O. Box 20
   50 Winter Sport Lane
   Williston, VT 05495-0020
   (Telephone orders: 800-216-2522; fax orders: 802-864-7626)

Australia
   Blackwell Science Pty, Ltd.
   54 University Street
   Carlton, Victoria 3053
   (Telephone orders: 03-9347-0300; fax orders: 03-9349-3016)

Outside The Americas and Australia
   Blackwell Science, Ltd.
   c/o Marston Book Services, Ltd.
   P.O. Box 269
   Abingdon
   Oxon OX14 4YN
   England
   (Telephone orders: 44-01235-465500; fax orders: 44-01235-465555)

Acquisitions: Beverly Copland
Development: Amy Nuttbrock
Production: Debra Lally
Manufacturing: Lisa Flanagan
Marketing Manager: Kathleen Mulcahy
Cover design: Leslie Haimes
Typeset by SNP Best-set Typesetter Ltd., Hong-Kong
Printed and bound by Sheridan Books

Printed in United States of America
02 03 04 05 5 4 3 2 1

Library of Congress Cataloging-in-Publication Data
   Marinella, Mark A., 1967–
     PocketBrain of 50 unusual symptoms / by Mark A. Marinella.
        p. ; cm.
     ISBN 0-632-04698-8 (pbk.)
     1. Symptoms—Handbooks, manuals, etc.
     [DNLM: 1. Diagnosis—Handbooks. WB 39 M338p 2002]
   I. Title: Pocketbrain of fifty unusual symptoms. II. Title.
   RC69 .M365 2002
   616'.047—dc21

                                    2001007476

Dedication

This book is dedicated to the memory of my late father, Eugene, who was always my number one fan.

Acknowledgments

I wish to thank Miguel Parilo, MD, and Steven Burdette, MD, for their suggestions and thoughtful review of the manuscript.

Table of Contents

Table of Contents

Table of Contents

Foreword

"To study the phenomena of disease without books is to sail an uncharted sea, while to study books without patients is not to go to sea at all."

—*William Osler,* Books and Men

Many can reflect on medical school as an endless quest to devour tremendous amounts of information and assemble this data into a usable and practical knowledge base. For many, this is an overwhelming and daunting task. It is often not until the clinical years of training that one realizes its usefulness or importance. *Pocket Brain of 50 Unusual Symptoms* is an excellent example of how these fundamental skills are applied in clinical practice.

Dr. Marinella's text does not serve as a complete textbook of internal medicine, but rather as a guide to various, often unrecognized, symptoms in medicine. This book illustrates how the internist takes the chief complaint and is able to apply this knowledge base, reaching the difficult diagnosis. It is this skill that the practiced internist thrives on.

This book is structured in a concise, quick, and practical fashion, making it easy to read and reference. With 50 examples, the reader is confronted with challenging cases and engaging discussions.

As an accomplished clinical and academic hospital–based internist, Dr. Marinella continually emphasizes a cornerstone principle of internal medicine: development of broad differential diagnosis based on pattern recognition and clinical experience. This makes *Pocket Brain of 50 Unusual Symptoms* a terrific tool for the internal medicine clerk, resident, or practitioner.

Miguel A. Parilo, MD
Assistant Clinical Professor of Medicine
Wright State University School of Medicine
Dayton, Ohio

Preface

Obtaining an accurate history from the patient is truly the most important step in reaching a timely, accurate diagnosis. Despite the plethora of advanced diagnostic aids at our disposal, a well-obtained patient history remains the backbone of establishing a diagnosis. Many illnesses are characterized by similar non-specific symptoms such as chest pain, abdominal pain, headache, dizziness, fatigue, fever, and weight loss, to name a few. Indeed, there are numerous disease processes that can present with similar symptoms. It is often the nature of these symptoms and the presence of other symptoms, as well as physical examination findings, that enable the clinician to narrow the differential diagnosis.

However, in some cases the predominant symptom or an accompanying symptom may be quite unusual and may not be recognized by the clinician and, as a result, may be dismissed due to unfamiliarity. The purpose of this book is to present a variety of unusual or peculiar symptoms that the clinician may encounter. Some patients may volunteer such symptoms. However, as clinicians we often must "pry" additional symptoms out of our patients. As such, increasing one's knowledge of a few unusual symptoms may assist the clinician in constructing an accurate, thorough patient history. This work is not meant to be an exhaustive volume of bizarre and unusual symptoms. Instead, it represents a compendium of symptoms the author has learned from his patients, as well as some uncommon symptoms of common diseases encountered in clinical practice. I invite suggestions from readers on other unusual symptoms for future editions.

This work is meant to be concise and easy to read in a short time. Medical students and house officers will find this book useful not only for their clinical rotations but also for board examinations and increasing their overall knowledge base. Practicing physicians and physician extenders may also find this book useful to expand their diagnostic acumen. Above all, I hope that readers will be stimulated to hone their history-taking skills, which may, in turn, lead to the recognition of a patient's illness in a more expedient manner.

Mark A. Marinella, MD, F.A.C.P.
Dayton, Ohio

Blood in the Semen

Significance: Blood in the ejaculate, or hematospermia, is an alarming symptom that can have a variety of etiologies, but, in general, is a self-limited symptom, especially in younger men.

ETIOLOGY

Prostate biopsy
Prostatic calculi
Chronic prostatitis
Prostate cancer
Neoplasm of the seminal vesicle
Hypertension
Sexually transmitted diseases
Hemophilia
Anticoagulants
Testicular neoplasm
Unknown

DISCUSSION

Hematospermia refers to the presence of blood in the ejaculate and often leads to immense emotional distress.

Hematospermia may result from inflammatory, infectious, neoplastic, systemic, or iatrogenic conditions, although many cases are idiopathic. Hematospermia results when blood enters the semen from the sexual glands (e.g., prostate, seminal vesicles), urethra, or bladder. Many studies reveal prostatic disease to be the most common etiology of hematospermia, although prostatic biopsy is considered the most common etiology overall. Prostatic calculi may account for 20% of cases of hematospermia and chronic prostatitis for up to 13% of cases. Miscellaneous structural etiologies include vascular malformations, benign and malignant testicular tumors, and cysts. Medical or systemic diseases are uncommon etiologies of hematospermia, the most common being uncontrolled hypertension and bleeding diastheses. Patients under 40 years of age are more likely to have an inflammatory cause for hematospermia, although many cases remain idiopathic. However, older men have an increased incidence of prostatic malignancy as an etiology of hematospermia. Evaluation of hematospermia includes a meticulous genitourinary and prostatic examination with judicious use of laboratory and radiologic tests. Most patients should undergo urinalysis and culture, semen analysis, and, if the patient is over 50 years of age, a serum prostate-specific antigen (PSA). Prostatic ultrasound, magnetic resonance imaging, cystoscopy, or prostatic biopsy may be necessary in some patients. Therapy of hematospermia may consist of reassurance in the young man with idiopathic hematospermia and treatment of underlying prostatitis or prostatic malignancy in older men.

ADDITIONAL READING

1. **Munkelwitz R, Krasnokutsky S, Lie J, et al.** Current perspectives on hematospermia: a review. J Androl 1997;18:6.
2. **Papp GK, Hoznek A, Hegedus M, et al.** Hematospermia. J Androl 1994;15:31S.

2

Burning and Redness of the Feet

Significance: Severe burning pain accompanied by redness and warmth that involves the feet is characteristic of erythromelalgia, an unusual disorder occasionally associated with various myeloproliferative disorders.

ETIOLOGY

Primary (idiopathic) form
Secondary form
   Essential thrombocythemia
   Polycythemia vera
   Chronic myelogenous leukemia
   Myeloid metaplasia
   Rheumatoid arthritis
   Lupus
   Vasculitis
   Other

DISCUSSION

Erthyromelalgia is an uncommon syndrome consisting of burning pain, erythema, and warmth that typically affects the feet and, less commonly, the hands. Primary or idiopathic erythromelalgia accounts for approximately half the cases with the remaining cases occurring in association with an underlying disease, usually a myeloproliferative disorder. Secondary erythromelalgia is more common in men and usually occurs during the sixth decade. Most cases of secondary erythromelalgia are associated with polycythemia vera or essential thrombocythemia. Intravascular clumping of platelets within arterioles with release of prostaglandins has been proposed as a pathophysiologic mechanism of erythromelalgia. Symptoms may predate diagnosis of a myeloproliferative syndrome by months or years. Symptoms usually involve the feet and consist of severe burning pain, throbbing, redness, and warmth and may be induced by limb dependency, exercise, and heat. Symptoms are usually relieved by elevation and cooling of the extremity or by administration of aspirin. Although diagnosis of erythromelalgia is clinical, a complete blood count should be obtained periodically to assess for evidence of a myeloproliferative disorder. Aspirin therapy may effectively control symptoms in many patients with erythromelalgia, although primary therapy for an underlying myeloproliferative disorder is essential in selected patients.

ADDITIONAL READING

1. **Kurzrock R, Cohen PR.** Erythromelalgia: review of clinical characteristics and pathophysiology. Am J Med 1991;91:416.
2. **Kurzrock R, Cohen PR.** Erythromelalgia and myeloproliferative disorders. Arch Intern Med 1989;149:105.

Coughing Up a "Stone"

Significance: Coughing up a stone, also known as lithoptysis, was first described by Aristotle and is a characteristic symptom of broncholithiasis.

ETIOLOGY

Histoplasmosis
Tuberculosis
Cryptococcosis
Coccidioidomycosis
Actinomycosis
Nocardiosis
Aspergillosis
Silicosis

DISCUSSION

Lithoptysis is an uncommon symptom that literally means to "cough up a stone." First described by Aristotle in 300 B.C., lithoptysis is indicative of the presence of broncholiths, which are calcified peribronchial lymph nodes that erode into the bronchial tree. Broncholiths are usually composed of calcium phosphate or calcium carbonate. In the setting of a pulmonary infection, most commonly histoplasmosis, the lung parenchyma becomes alkaline, which enhances local precipitation of calcium phosphate and carbonate. Rarely, patients with other fungal lung infections or silicosis may develop broncholiths. These calcifications typically form in the peribronchial lymph nodes and are usually asymptomatic unless one erodes into the airway lumen and is expectorated. In addition to lithoptysis, broncholithiasis may lead to cough, sputum production, hemoptysis, and recurrent episodes of post-obstructive pneumonia. Patients with lithoptysis may note gritty or sandy sputum or may actually cough up a small, stonelike object, which is pathognomonic for broncholithiasis. Rare complications of broncholithiasis include bronchoesophageal, aortoesophageal, aortotracheal, or bronchopleural fistula formation. Diagnosis of broncholithiasis is mainly clinical, especially if the patient saves the stone and presents it to the physician for analysis. Chest radiography, computed tomography, and bronchoscopy are useful for confirming the diagnosis and excluding complications. Treatment of patients with lithoptysis is generally supportive, although antibiotics are indicated for postobstructive pneumonia, and surgery may be needed if a complication is present.

ADDITIONAL READING

1. **Haines JD.** Coughing up a stone: what to do about broncholithiasis. Postgrad Med 1988;83:83.
2. **Samson IM, Rossoff LJ.** Chronic lithoptysis with multiple bilateral broncholiths. Chest 1997;112:563.

4

Coughing up Sputum That Settles into Three Layers

Significance: Copious purulent sputum production that settles into three layers when expectorated into a receptacle is characteristic of bronchiectasis.

ETIOLOGY

Bronchiectasis
    Prior lung infection (e.g., prior necrotizing pneumonia, viral, fungal)
    Cystic fibrosis
    Alpha-1-antitrypsin deficiency
    Inhalation injury
    Kartagener's syndrome
    Hypogammaglobulinemia
    Congenital

DISCUSSION

The chronic production of excessive purulent, foul-smelling sputum that settles into three layers is characteristic of bronchiectasis. Bronchiectasis is defined as permanent bronchial dilatation resulting from destructive inflammatory changes within the elastic and muscular walls of the bronchi. Bronchiectasis may be confined to one lung segment or be diffuse in nature, affecting most portions of the lungs. The most common etiologies of bronchiectasis are prior pulmonary infection with various viruses or bacteria that result in significant bronchial destruction. Other noninfectious etiologies may be responsible as well. As a result of chronic inflammation and bronchial damage, the mucociliary clearance mechanisms of the lung are affected, which leads to pooling of excess secretions that then become secondarily infected, resulting in increased purulent sputum production. Patients with bronchiectasis not uncommonly present during adulthood with chronic cough, hemoptysis, fever, and weight loss that result from chronic bacterial superinfection, often with Gram-negative bacteria. The classic symptom is copious production of purulent, foul-smelling sputum that may approach volumes of 500 cc per day. A characteristic, but uncommon, symptom of bronchiectasis is patients' reporting that their sputum settles into three distinct layers if they expectorate it into a cup or other receptacle. The three layers consist of a frothy top layer that consists of watery saliva; a middle mucoid layer consisting of glandular mucus; and a bottom purulent layer. Patients suspected of having bronchiectasis based on history should undergo chest radiography and, if indicated, high-resolution computed tomographic scanning of the chest to assess the severity. Antimicrobial therapy is often administered to control acute infectious exacerbations in patients with bronchiectasis, although some patients may require chronic suppressive therapy.

ADDITIONAL READING

1. **Mysliwiec V, Pina JS.** Bronchiectasis: the other obstructive lung disease. Postgrad Med 1999;106;123.

2. **Scharf SM.** Laboratory evaluation of patients with respiratory disease. In: Textbook of pulmonary diseases. Baum GL, Wolinsky E, eds. 4th ed. Boston: Little, Brown and Company, 1989:227–241.

Coughing up Pink, Frothy Sputum

Significance: The complaint of pink, frothy sputum, in conjunction with acute dyspnea, is characteristic of acute pulmonary edema.

ETIOLOGY

Cardiogenic pulmonary edema
    Cardiac ischemia
    Cardiomyopathy
    Uncontrolled hypertension
    Valvular disease
    Volume overload
Noncardiogenic pulmonary edema
    Opiates
    Head injury
    High-altitude sickness
    Aspiration
    Inhalational injury

DISCUSSION

The symptom of pink, frothy sputum, as well as acute dyspnea, is characteristic of acute pulmonary edema.

Acute pulmonary edema may be cardiogenic or noncardiogenic in origin. Acute cardiogenic pulmonary edema is more common and is typically caused by an exacerbation of congestive heart failure. When the left atrial pressure acutely rises as a result of an increase in left ventricular end-diastolic pressure and volume, a concurrent increase in pulmonary venous and capillary pressure occurs. When an increase in the capillary hydrostatic pressure above a critical level occurs, there is a net increase in fluid filtration into the interstitial and, eventually, the alveolar space. Noncardiogenic pulmonary edema occurs in the presence of "leaky" alveolar capillaries (e.g., aspiration, drug ingestion, head injury, etc.), which leads to rapid fluid collection within the alveolar space. Symptoms of acute pulmonary edema include the sudden onset of fear, anxiety, hyperventilation, and severe air hunger. The clinical picture is quite characteristic, with the patient sitting up, pale, diaphoretic, and anxious. A classic symptom usually associated with acute cardiogenic pulmonary edema is the production of copious, pink, frothy sputum, which results from capillary rupture due to the increased hydrostatic pressure. Patients may be quite startled with this symptom and bring it to the clinician's attention quickly. Confirmation of pulmonary edema can usually be made by physical examination and a chest radiograph. Further investigations should be based on the likely etiology. Loop diuretics, nitrates, oxygen, and morphine are typically used to treat acute cardiogenic pulmonary edema; other less common etiologies often require supportive therapy.

ADDITIONAL READING

1. **Angerio AD, Kot PA.** Pathophysiology of acute pulmonary edema. Crit Care Nurs Q 1994;17:21.
2. **Jacobson ND.** Acute high-altitude illness. Am Fam Physician 1988;38:135.

Craving and Eating Large Amounts of Ice

Significance: The symptom of craving and ingesting large amounts of ice, a form of pica known as pagophagia, is a common manifestation of iron deficiency anemia.

ETIOLOGY

Iron deficiency anemia
  Gastrointestinal blood loss
  Menstrual blood loss
  Chronic hematuria

DISCUSSION

Pica, the abnormal craving for unusual types of food or nonnutritive substances, is an occasional manifestation of iron deficiency anemia. Patients may ingest large amounts of salty or crunchy foods such as pretzels, carrots, celery, or lettuce. Some patients may ingest tomatoes, dirt, clay, or other inert substances such as starch. Children with iron deficiency anemia have been reported to ingest dirt (geophagia), which may result in lead poisoning if lead paint chips are present in the soil. Pica occurs in approximately 50% of patients with iron deficiency anemia. Pagophagia is a form of pica characterized by the abnormal craving and ingestion of ice and is by far the most common type of pica in patients with iron deficiency anemia. Pagophagia usually results from iron deficiency resulting from chronic gastrointestinal blood loss. Many patients will not volunteer the information that they ingest large amounts of ice. As such, the clinician should inquire about this symptom if other symptoms and signs of iron deficiency are present. Determination of serum hemoglobin and iron studies should be performed in patients with pagophagia and other types of pica. Treatment of iron deficiency anemia with iron preparations should result in normalization of the hematocrit and resolution of pica.

ADDITIONAL READING

1. **Marinella MA.** "Tomatophagia" and iron deficiency anemia. N Engl J Med 1999;341:60.
2. **Rector WG.** Pica: its frequency and significance in patients with iron deficiency anemia due to chronic gastrointestinal blood loss. J Gen Intern Med 1989;4:512.

7

Craving Ice Water

Significance: Intense thirst with the craving for ice-cold water is an occasional symptom of diabetes insipidus.

ETIOLOGY

Diabetes insipidus
    Central
    Nephrogenic

DISCUSSION

Diabetes insipidus results from lack of vasopressin (central diabetes insipidus) or renal tubular resistance to vasopressin (nephrogenic diabetes insipidus). Deficiency of vasopressin or renal resistance to vasopressin leads to enhanced renal water loss, which can lead to cardiovascular collapse and hypernatremia if the patient cannot replenish water losses. Central diabetes insipidus may be idiopathic or result from structural damage to the hypothalamus from metastatic tumors, infection, granulomatous diseases, head trauma, and neurosurgical procedures. Nephrogenic diabetes insipidus may be inherited as an X-linked trait or, more commonly, result from various drugs (e.g., lithium), prolonged urinary tract obstruction, myeloma, sickle cell anemia, and electrolyte abnormalities. The characteristic clinical picture of diabetes insipidus consists of significant passage of hypotonic urine (up to 20 liters per day) and polydypsia. Patients with diabetes insipidus also commonly complain of intense thirst and may crave ice-cold water, which may be a helpful clue to the diagnosis. Patients suspected of having diabetes insipidus should have their serum electrolytes measured and, if possible, undergo a water-deprivation test if the diagnosis is in question. Treatment of central diabetes insipidus consists of synthetic vasopressin administration (DDAVP, desargine des-amino vasopressin). Treatment of nephrogenic diabetes insipidus may be more difficult, although thiazide diuretics may benefit some patients.

ADDITIONAL READING

1. **Bichet DG.** Nephrogenic diabetes insipidus. Am J Med 1998; 105:431.
2. **Seckl JR, Dunger DB.** Diabetes insipidus: current treatment recommendations. Drugs 1992;44:216.

8

Craving Salt

Significance: The craving of salt and salty foods is a characteristic symptom of Addison's disease.

ETIOLOGY

Addison's disease
  Autoimmune
  Tuberculosis
  Histoplasmosis
  Adrenal hemorrhage
  Metastatic adrenal lesions
  Amyloidosis
  Adrenal infarction

DISCUSSION

The symptom of craving salt is a helpful clue to the diagnosis of Addison's disease. Addison's disease, primary adrenal failure, results from destruction of the adrenal gland cortex, usually due to an autoimmune etiology, although several other etiologies have been reported. Loss of the adrenal cortex notably results in hypocortisolism and mineralocorticoid deficiency, both of which cause the myriad of signs and symptoms associated with Addison's disease. Patients with Addison's disease may present with a variety of nonspecific symptoms such as malaise, orthostatic dizziness, anorexia, weight loss, nausea, and depression. Since mineralocorticoid deficiency is present, abnormalities in sodium homeostasis are common, leading to the characteristic volume contraction and postural hypotension associated with this disorder. Salt craving is a distinctive symptom of Addison's disease and likely results from aldosterone deficiency, which leads to natriuresis and sodium depletion. Patients may crave salt or very salty foods such as pretzels or potato chips. Some patients may ingest very large quantities of sodium to satisfy their craving. For unclear reasons, some patients "chase" their salt ingestion with lemon juice. Patients suspected of having Addison's disease should undergo electrolyte analysis and have an ACTH stimulation test performed. Addison's disease is fatal if untreated and timely replacement with supplemental hydrocortisone is necessary.

ADDITIONAL READING

1. **Davenport J, Kellerman C, Reiss D, et al.** Addison's disease. Am Fam Physician 1991;43:1338.
2. **Orth DN, Kovacs WJ.** The adrenal cortex. In: Williams' Textbook of endocrinology. 9th ed. Philadelphia: W.B. Saunders, 1998:517–664.

Difficulty in Releasing a Handshake

Significance: The symptom of difficulty releasing a hand-grip, as in a handshake, suggests impaired muscle relaxation known as myotonia, which is a common feature of myotonic disorders.

ETIOLOGY

Myotonic dystrophy
Myotonia congenita
Chondrodystrophic myotonia

DISCUSSION

Difficulty in releasing the grip of an object or a handshake is a peculiar symptom known as myotonia and is a hallmark of myotonic dystrophy and other less common myotonias. Myotonia is a prominent feature of the autosomal dominant disorder myotonic dystrophy, which is characterized by muscle atrophy, weakness, cardiac abnormalities, cataracts, baldness, and testicular atrophy in males. In addition, myotonia is the predominant manifestation of the autosomal-dominant disorder myotonia congenita, which does not cause systemic disorders as does myotonic dystrophy. Myotonia is often most evident in the hands. Patients with myotonia of any etiology typically note symptoms of difficulty releasing a handgrip. For instance, it may be very difficult, as well as embarrassing, for the patient to release from a handshake or to let go of an object such as a doorknob. Myotonia can often be elicited by shaking the patient's hand or by tapping on the muscles of the forearm, which reveals slow relaxation of muscle contraction. Diagnosis of myotonic dystrophy is suggested by the presence of the systemic findings as noted above. Myotonia has characteristic electromyographic findings such as continuous high-frequency muscle discharge after relaxation ensues. There is no specific therapy for myotonic dystrophy other than supportive, symptomatic care.

ADDITIONAL READING

1. **Ashizawa T.** Myotonic dystrophy as a brain disorder. Arch Neurol 1998;55:291.
2. **Thornton CA, Ashizawa T.** Getting a grip on the myotonic dystrophies. Neurology 1999;52:12.

10

Discharge from the Nipples Resembling Milk

Significance: Discharge of milk from the nipples in a non-lactating woman or a man, known as galactorrhea, typically signifies hyperprolactinemia.

ETIOLOGY

Prolactinoma
Drugs (e.g., phenothiazines, estrogens, cimetidine, haloperidol, narcotics)
Cirrhosis
Chest wall stimulation or irritation
Thoracotomy
Herpes zoster
Mastectomy
Nipple rings
Chronic renal failure
Severe stress
Ectopic prolactin production by malignancy (e.g., lung cancer, renal cell carcinoma)
Pituitary stalk damage (e.g., surgery, tumor, trauma)

DISCUSSION

Discharge of breast milk from a man or a nonpregnant woman is known as galactorrhea and is usually indicative of hyperprolactinemia. Prolactin is normally secreted by the lactotroph cells of the anterior pituitary gland and mainly serves to stimulate milk production from the mammary glands. Increased levels of prolactin classically cause galactorrhea, which should lead to evaluation if the patient is nonpregnant or male. In addition, trauma or section of the pituitary stalk may lead to galactorrhea through interruption of the tonic hormone dopamine, which suppresses prolactin secretion. There are many etiologies of hyperprolactinemia. However, a pituitary adenoma always needs to be considered and should be excluded if the patient has no other obvious etiology such as certain medications, chest wall irritation, or cirrhosis. Headache or visual disturbance should suggest a pituitary adenoma. The classic symptom of hyperprolactinemia, regardless of etiology, is galactorrhea or discharge of milk from the nipples. Patients may note the actual dribbling of milk or note stains on their shirt or bra. The discharge is usually white, although it may be yellow-tinged. Patients with galactorrhea should undergo careful review of their medications, as well as visual field testing if there is concern for a large pituitary adenoma. Serum prolactin measurement is essential as is magnetic resonance imaging of the sella if a pituitary adenoma is suspected. Treatment of prolactinoma often consists of bromocriptine, although some patients require surgical resection of the tumor.

ADDITIONAL READING

1. **Conner P, Fried G.** Hyperprolactinemia: etiology, diagnosis, and treatment alternatives. Acta Obstet Gynecol Scand 1998;77: 249.
2. **Luciano AA.** Clinical presentation of hyperprolactinemia. J Reprod Med 1999;44:1085.

11

Dyspnea Occurring at Night with Need to Seek Fresh Air

Significance: Severe dyspnea awakening the patient from sleep and causing a smothering sensation is a classic symptom of left ventricular failure.

ETIOLOGY

Left-sided congestive heart failure
Transient myocardial ischemia
Critical aortic stenosis

DISCUSSION

The sudden onset of nocturnal breathlessness, paroxysmal nocturnal dyspnea, is a very characteristic symptom of left-sided heart failure or myocardial ischemia. The patho-physiology of paroxysmal nocturnal dyspnea is not fully elucidated, but is it likely caused by increased thoracic blood volume resulting from recumbency, decreased nocturnal adrenergic drive to the ventricle, and nocturnal depression of the respiratory center. In addition, transient myocardial ischemia may result in decreased compliance of the ventricle leading to an abrupt increase in left-ventricular end-diastolic pressure. Symptoms of paroxysmal nocturnal dyspnea may occur nightly or only sporadically. The patient is typically awakened approximately 2 hours after falling asleep with severe dyspnea and a smothering sensation that may be accompanied by cough and severe anxiety or a sense of impending doom. The dyspnea is not typically relieved by sitting up in bed, and the patient typically needs to stand up and seek fresh air by opening a window or turning on a fan to obtain relief. The symptoms usually last 15 to 30 minutes before subsiding. Patients with paroxysmal nocturnal dyspnea should undergo assessment for evidence of depressed left ventricular function, as well as myocardial ischemia. Treatment of paroxysmal nocturnal dyspnea includes optimizing cardiac function with vasodilators, beta-blockers, nitrates, diuretics, and revascularization, if indicated.

ADDITIONAL READING

1. **Burch GE.** Of paroxysmal nocturnal dyspnea. Am Heart J 1979;98:812.
2. **Fuster V.** The clinical history. In: Cardiology: fundamentals and practice. 2nd ed. Guiliani ER, Fuster V, Gersh BJ, et al., eds. St. Louis: Mosby–Year Book, 1991:189–203.

12

Dyspnea While Lying on One's Side

Significance: Dyspnea in the lateral decubitus position, also known as trepopnea, may occur with a variety of cardiopulmonary conditions.

ETIOLOGY

Pleural effusion
Congestive heart failure
Endobronchial malignancy
Atrial septal defect
Atrial myxoma
Tumor growth into the right atrium
   Renal cell carcinoma
   Hepatocellular carcinoma

DISCUSSION

Trepopnea is the symptom of dyspnea when the patient assumes the lateral recumbent position. Patients may note dyspnea when lying on their left or right side, which is relieved by changing body position. There are several etiologies of trepopnea, but most cases result from cardiopulmonary disease. For instance, in cases of pleural effusion or endobronchial obstruction, dyspnea results from increased gravitational perfusion of a lung that is poorly ventilated. Some authors contend that trepopnea results from an enlarged heart compressing the pulmonary veins when the patient lies on their side. Trepopnea may also occur in the presence of arteriovenous malformations of the lung that are preferentially perfused in the lateral recumbent position, resulting in a transient right-to-left shunt. Cases of right-sided trepopnea have been reported in patients with atrial septal defects due to the weight of the heart pulling down the septum causing increased blood flow through the defect. Assessment of patients with trepopnea should include a thorough physical examination, a chest radiograph, and, if evidence of significant heart disease is present, an echocardiogram. Selected patients may need bronchoscopy to exclude an endobronchial lesion. Treatment of the patient with trepopnea is directed at the underlying etiology, but may include thoracentesis if a large pleural effusion is present or maximizing therapy for heart failure.

ADDITIONAL READING

1. **Alfaifi S, Lapinsky SE**. Trepopnea due to interatrial shunt following lung resection. Chest 1998;113:1726.
2. **Wise JR**. Trepopnea. N Engl J Med 1970;282:266.

13

Dyspnea in the Standing Position

Significance: Dyspnea occurring in the standing position that is relieved in the supine position is known as platypnea and usually results from enhanced gravitational blood flow through pulmonary arteriovenous malformations or an atrial septal defect.

ETIOLOGY

Pulmonary arteriovenous malformations
   Hepatopulmonary syndrome
   Osler-Weber-Rendu disease
   Congenital
Atrial septal defect
Pleural effusion
Multiple pulmonary emboli
Severe obstructive lung disease

DISCUSSION

Platypnea is an unusual symptom that consists of dyspnea in the upright position that is relieved in the recumbent position. Platypnea is characteristically accompanied by orthodeoxia, a decrease in oxygen saturation and PO_2 that occurs in the upright position ("platypnea-orthodeoxia syndrome"). Patients with pulmonary arteriovenous malformations due to cirrhosis-induced hepatopulmonary syndrome, Osler-Weber-Rendu disease, and congenital etiologies frequently develop platypnea. The mechanism for platypnea-orthodeoxia in these patients likely results from increased gravitational blood flow through the basal lung segments, leading to increased right-to-left shunt and arterial hypoxemia. Cases of platypnea-orthodeoxia syndrome have been reported in patients with obstructive lung disease and pleural effusions, which likely result from increased ventilation-perfusion (VQ) mismatch. Patent foramen ovale occasionally leads to platypnea-orthodeoxia, possibly by increased blood flow from a noncompliant right atrium into a compliant left atrium. Diagnosis of platypnea-orthodeoxia is mainly by history and measurement of arterial oxygen levels in the supine and erect positions. Ventilation-perfusion nuclear scanning reveals increased tracer uptake in the brain and kidneys in cases of pulmonary arteriovenous malformations. If a patent foramen ovale is suspected, a bubble-contrast echocardiogram is a helpful diagnostic aid. Treatment of platypnea is difficult in the patient with hepatopulmonary syndrome, but liver transplantation may ameliorate the symptoms. Angiographic embolization of pulmonary arteriovenous malformations may be effective in patients with Osler-Weber-Rendu disease.

ADDITIONAL READING

1. **Malbrain MLNG, Brans B, Lambrecht GLY**. Platypnea-orthodeoxia syndrome. Acta Cardiologica 1995;50:103.
2. **Robin ED, McCauley RF**. An analysis of platypnea-orthodeoxia syndrome including a "new" therapeutic approach. Chest 1997;112:1449.

Electric Shock–Like Sensation with Neck Flexion

Significance: An electric-shock sensation that radiates down the spine and legs on flexion of the neck is known as Lhermitte's symptom, which often signifies significant spinal cord pathology.

ETIOLOGY

Multiple sclerosis
Vitamin B12 deficiency
Cervical spondylosis
Spinal cord tumor
Previous radiotherapy
Head and neck trauma
Vascular malformation of the spinal cord
Systemic lupus erythematosus
Chemotherapy
  Cisplatinum
  Docetaxel

DISCUSSION

Lhermitte's symptom, the sensation of an electric shock radiating along the spinal column and lower limbs on neck flexion, was reported by Jean Lhermitte in 1924. Lhermitte, a French physician, presented the sentinel report of the symptom to the Neurological Society of Paris in 1924, entitled "Pain of an Electric Discharge Character Following Head Flexion in Multiple Sclerosis." The symptom occurred in a young woman with multiple sclerosis and was described as follows: "upon bending of the head, a violent shock in the neck and a pain resembling an electric current which traveled the body from the neck to the feet." The symptom likely results from demyelination of the cervical spinal cord and classically occurs with multiple sclerosis, which is characterized by demyelinization of central nervous tissue. Many other etiologies, as noted above, have been associated with Lhermitte's symptom as well and result from damage to myelin within the spinal cord, notably the posterior columns. Patients with Lhermitte's symptom should have a careful history obtained, with special attention to other symptoms of multiple sclerosis or prior administration of radiotherapy or chemotherapy. In addition to a thorough neurologic examination, magnetic resonance imaging of the brain and cervical spinal cord should be considered. Treatment depends on the etiology.

ADDITIONAL READING

1. **Lewanski CR, Sinclair JA, Stewart JS.** Lhermitte's sign following head and neck radiotherapy. Clinical Oncol 2000;12:98.
2. **Gutrecht JA.** Lhermitte's sign: from observation to eponym. Arch Neurol 1989;46:557.

15

Fear of Drinking Water

Significance: Fear of ingesting fluids, hydrophobia, is a characteristic symptom of rabies, a fatal zoonotic illness of the central nervous system.

ETIOLOGY

Rabies from various animals
  Bat
  Bobcat
  Coyote
  Dog
  Fox
  Livestock
  Raccoon
  Skunk
  Woodchuck

DISCUSSION

Rabies is a zoonotic viral infection acquired from the bite or scratch of a mammal infected with the rabies virus. Worldwide, rabid dogs are the most common mode of transmission of rabies to humans. However, in the United States, other mammals such as bats, skunks, and raccoons are more commonly associated with the transmission of rabies. The rabies virus is a bullet-shaped RNA virus that travels along peripheral nerves to the central nervous system. The incubation period of rabies ranges from 20 to 90 days after which the patient develops various non-specific symptoms, including confusion, fever, and abdominal discomfort. After several days, many patients develop involuntary spasms of the pharyngeal muscles precipitated by drinking water (hydrophobia), which is pathognomonic for rabies infection. The muscle spasms may also involve the diaphragm and the sternocleidomastoid muscles. The spasms create intense terror and anxiety for the patient and are very alarming to onlookers. In addition to the ingestion of water, the sight, sound, or even mention of water may involve significant muscle spasms. Diagnosis of rabies can be made with a biopsy of the nape of the neck, although the characteristic histologic finding is the presence of Negri bodies on brain biopsy or autopsy specimens. There is no effective therapy for full-blown rabies, with most patients dying within days of developing hydrophobia.

ADDITIONAL READING

1. **Murphy FA.** Rabies pathogenesis. Arch Virol 1977;54:279.
2. **Warrell DA.** The clinical picture of rabies in man. Trans R Soc Trop Med Hyg 1976;70:188.

16

Fear of Eating

Significance: Fear of eating, sitophobia, is a classic symptom of chronic mesenteric vascular ischemia.

ETIOLOGY

Chronic mesenteric ischemia
   Atherosclerotic (>90% of cases)
   Fibromuscular dysplasia
   Vasculitis

DISCUSSION

Fear of eating (sitophobia) is a characteristic symptom of chronic mesenteric artery ischemia. Chronic mesenteric arterial ischemia typically results when significant atherosclerotic narrowing of the celiac and superior mesenteric vessels is present. Rare cases are due to fibromuscular dysplasia or vasculitis. Occlusion of these arteries leads to decreased blood flow to the intestines when increased metabolic demand is present, as occurs after eating. Decreased flow postprandially leads to mucosal ischemia, which may result in nutrient malabsorption and weight loss. Typical symptoms of chronic mesenteric ischemia consist of epigastric or periumbilical abdominal pain that begins approximately 30 to 60 minutes after eating (intestinal angina). The pain is usually constant and crampy in nature and may last up to 3 hours. A characteristic symptom of chronic mesenteric ischemia, however, is a fear of eating or aversion to food. Patients may be afraid to eat because food ingestion typically leads to significant postprandial pain. As a result, weight loss is present in most patients with chronic mesenteric ischemia. In fact, pain that persists during the fasting state should lead to consideration of other diagnoses. Patients suspected of having chronic mesenteric ischemia should undergo visceral angiography. Patients with atherosclerotic mesenteric ischemia should stop smoking and receive intense therapy for diabetes, hypertension, and hyperlipidemia. Some patients require arterial angioplasty or surgical revascularization.

ADDITIONAL READING

1. **Moawad J, Gewertz BL.** Chronic mesenteric ischemia. Surg Clin North Am 1997;77:357.
2. **Reiner L.** Mesenteric arterial insufficiency and abdominal angina. Arch Intern Med 1964;114:765.

Headache After Eating a Protein-Rich Meal

Significance: Migraine-like headaches after protein consumption are a frequent manifestation of ornithine transcarbamylase deficiency.

ETIOLOGY

Ornithine transcarbamylase deficiency

DISCUSSION

Deficiency of the enzyme ornithine transcarbamylase results in elevated serum ammonia levels. Ornithine transcarbamylase, an enzyme present in Krebs' cycle, catalyzes the formation of citrulline from carbamyl phosphate and ornithine. Deficiency of ornithine transcarbamylase results in accumulation of orotic acid, which is excreted in the urine. In addition, elevated serum ammonia levels occur, resulting in neurologic dysfunction. Ornithine transcarbamylase deficiency is inherited as an X-linked recessive trait, which usually results in severe illness and death in male neonates. Carrier females, however, may not develop symptoms until early adulthood. Symptoms of adult-onset ornithine transcarbamylase deficiency typically occur after a protein-rich meal (such as meat or poultry) and include confusion, nausea, vomiting, and lethargy. A classic symptom occurring in carriers, however, is a migraine-like headache that follows ingestion of protein. As such, patients with a severe headache or confusion after protein consumption should undergo metabolic evaluation to exclude ornithine transcarbamylase deficiency. Serum ammonia is typically elevated in such patients and serves as a simple screening test for this disorder. In addition, serum citrulline levels are depressed and serum and urine orotic acid levels are elevated. Treatment options include amino acid supplementation and limitation of dietary protein.

ADDITIONAL READING

1. **DiMagno EP, Lowe JE, Snodgrass PJ, et al.** Ornithine transcarbamylase deficiency: a cause of bizarre behavior in a man. N Engl J Med 1986;315:744.
2. **Gilchrist JM, Coleman RA.** Ornithine transcarbamylase deficiency: adult onset of severe symptoms. Ann Intern Med 1987;106:556.

18

Headache and Palpitations During Urination

Significance: Headache and palpitations that complicate urination are very suggestive of a bladder pheochromocytoma, a rare etiology of secondary hypertension.

ETIOLOGY

Pheochromocytoma of bladder

DISCUSSION

Headache, palpitations, and diaphoresis are the classic symptom triad of pheochromocytoma, and symptom onset during urination is very suggestive of pheochromocytoma of the urinary bladder. Irritation of the tumor by changes in vesicular pressure may induce release of catecholamines, which are responsible for the classic symptoms of pheochromocytoma. Symptoms of bladder pheochromocytoma include tremor, nausea, anxiety, paresthesias, visual blurring, dizziness, and a salty taste in the mouth, all of which occur during urination. Symptoms usually cease after several minutes. Rarely, symptoms have been reported to occur during insertion of a urinary catheter. Diagnosis of a bladder pheochromocytoma is based on recognizing the typical symptoms that occur during urination followed by biochemical confirmation of elevated levels of urinary catecholamines and their metabolites. Anatomical diagnosis is best performed via cystoscopy. Definitive treatment of bladder pheochromocytoma is surgical resection preceded by effective control of the hypertension with agents such as phentolamine.

ADDITIONAL READING

1. **Ludmerer KM, Kissane JM**. Micturation-induced hypertension in a 58-year-old woman. Am J Med 1985;78:307.
2. **Raper AJ, et al**. Pheochromocytoma of the urinary bladder: a broad clinical spectrum. Am J Cardiol 1977;40:820.

19

Headache During an Orgasm

Significance: A severe headache occurring during an orgasm is usually a benign headache syndrome (benign orgasmic cephalgia), although subarachnoid hemorrhage may also present in this manner.

ETIOLOGY

Benign orgasmic cephalgia
Subarachnoid hemorrhage
Leaking Berry aneurysm ("sentinel bleed")
Intraparenchymal brain hemorrhage

DISCUSSION

A severe headache occurring during an orgasm is a very alarming symptom that is usually self-limited, although few patients may have significant intracranial pathology. The term "benign orgasmic cephalgia" has been applied to headaches that occur during sexual intercourse or to a severe, acute headache at the time of orgasm. Headaches occurring during the act of intercourse may result from sustained contraction of the cervical and scalp musculature. However, the more impressive type of coital headache occurs at the height of orgasm and may simulate a ruptured intracranial aneurysm. This type of headache (benign orgasmic cephalgia) may be retro-orbital, occipital, or global. The pain is throbbing and very intense. The etiology of pain may be due to vascular spasm or a low spinal fluid pressure from an occult tear in the subarachnoid membrane that occurs during intercourse. Orgasmic cephalgia predominates in men and may be recurrent, but is without sequelae. However, rare patients may experience a severe headache during coitus that is due to a ruptured Berry aneursym or a bleeding arteriovenous malformation. Patients with subarachnoid hemorrhage, however, may also experience nausea, vomiting, and clouding of sensorium. Patients presenting with severe headache during sexual intercourse should undergo computed tomography of the brain and possibly lumbar puncture or angiography if subarachnoid hemorrhage cannot be excluded. Treatment of benign orgasmic cephalgia is symptomatic, with provision of analgesic agents if necessary.

ADDITIONAL READING

1. **Dalessio DJ.** Headache and arterial hypertension. In: Wolff's Headache and other head pain. Dalessio DJ, ed. New York: Oxford University Press, 1980:184–197.
2. **Paulson GW, Klawans HL.** Benign orgasmic cephalgia. Headache 1974;13:181.

20

Hot and Cold Temperature Reversal

Significance: Temperature reversal, manifested as cold objects feeling hot and hot objects feeling cold, is a characteristic symptom of ciguatera fish poisoning, which results from ingestion of marine fish contaminated with dinoflagellate toxins.

ETIOLOGY

Ingestion of fish species including:
Amberjack
Anchovy
Barracuda
Bonito
Eel
Grouper
Sea bass
Snapper

DISCUSSION

Ciguatera fish poisoning is an underrecognized illness resulting from ingestion of ocean fish contaminated with toxins known collectively as ciguatoxin. Ciguatoxin is produced by a variety of dinoflagellates, eukaryotic marine organisms that attach to algae and large reef systems. Many species of fish consume algae-containing dinoflagellates. Larger carnivorous fish, in turn, ingest smaller fish and the ciguatoxin concentrates within the tissues of the fish, which leads to human illness when ingested. Ciguatoxin is an odorless, colorless, tasteless, heat-stable toxin that results in the inhibition of calcium regulation of the sodium channel. Affected fish usually taste normal, but may have a "peppery" taste. Symptoms usually occur within 3 hours of ingestion and include nausea, vomiting, diarrhea, and abdominal cramping. Neurologic symptoms, however, are quite common and are helpful clues to the diagnosis. Nonspecific symptoms such as paresthesias and dizziness commonly occur, but the characteristic, if not pathognomonic, symptom of ciguatera fish poisoning is temperature reversal. Patients may note that warm environments feel cold and cold environments feel hot. In addition, cold objects may feel warm or hot, and vice versa. Serious burns have been reported when patients touched a hot object they perceived as cold. Diagnosis of ciguatera fish poisoning is clinical, and any patient with gastrointestinal symptoms and cold-hot temperature reversal should be questioned about recent seafood ingestion. Treatment of ciguatera fish poisoning is mainly supportive and may include antihistamines and intravenous fluids.

ADDITIONAL READING

1. **Morris JG.** Ciguatera fish poisoning: barracuda's revenge. South Med J 1990;83:371.
2. **Withers NW.** Ciguatera fish poisoning. Ann Rev Med 1982; 33:97.

Increasing Hat, Glove, and Ring Size

Significance: Gradual enlargement of the head and hands leading to an increased hat and glove size is characteristic of acromegaly.

ETIOLOGY

Acromegaly
  Pituitary macroadenoma
  Pituitary carcinoma
  Carcinoid tumors
  Pancreatic tumors

DISCUSSION

Gradual enlargement of the skull, hands, and feet is characteristic of acromegaly, a syndrome of excess growth hormone secretion. Growth hormone, normally released by the pituitary gland, exerts its trophic effects via the hepatic release of insulin-like growth factor I (IGF-I). Pathologic increases in growth hormone before epiphyseal fusion results in gigantism. However, once bone growth is complete, excess growth hormone secretion results in increased appositional growth of bone and soft tissues, which leads to the characteristic manifestations of acromegaly. The vast majority of cases of acromegaly are due to a histologically benign pituitary macroadenoma. Rare cases result from a malignant pituitary tumor or excessive ectopic release of growth hormone. Weight gain, hypertension, osteoarthritis, a deepened voice, excessive perspiration, hyperglycemia, and carpal tunnel syndrome are frequent nonspecific manifestations of acromegaly. A characteristic symptom of acromegaly, however, is a gradual increase in hat size, which results from increased growth of the skull and surrounding soft tissues. Other characteristic symptoms include increasing glove, ring, and shoe size, which result from excessive bone and tissue growth of the hands and feet. Patients suspected of having acromegaly should undergo a magnetic resonance imaging scan to search for a pituitary adenoma. Serum IGF-1 and growth hormone levels should also be measured to confirm the diagnosis. Treatment of acromegaly includes surgical resection of the tumor and bromocriptine.

ADDITIONAL READING

1. **Barkan AL.** New options for diagnosing and treating acromegaly. Cleve Clin J Med 1998;65:343.
2. **Jaffe CA, Barkan AL.** Treatment of acromegaly with dopamine agonists. Endocrinol Metab Clin North Am 1992;21:713.

Laughing at Inappropriate Times

Significance: Laughing at inappropriate times and for no particular reason is an unusual, but quite characteristic, symptom of progressive supranuclear palsy and diseases associated with pseudobulbar palsy.

ETIOLOGY

Progressive supranuclear palsy
Pseudobulbar palsy
   Amyotrophic lateral sclerosis
   Multiple sclerosis
   Ischemic stroke

DISCUSSION

The inappropriate show of emotion, typically laughing or crying, is occasionally associated with serious central nervous system disease, classically, progressive supranuclear palsy (PSP) and amyotrophic lateral sclerosis (ALS). Atrophy of the midbrain, globus pallidus, and subthalamic nucleus is characteristic of PSP. These areas are characteristically infiltrated with neurofibrillary tangles, and neuronal loss is prominent. Patients with PSP often have bradykinesia similar to Parkinson's disease, but resting tremor is unusual. The characteristic clinical picture of PSP consists of ocular palsy (mainly vertical gaze), pseudobulbar palsy, rigidity, ataxia, and, eventually, subcortical dementia. An uncommon but useful clue is the symptom of inappropriate emotional lability, often manifested by outbursts of crying or laughter. Diagnosis of PSP is mainly clinical, and the diagnosis should be considered in any older patient with rigidity and gaze paresis, especially if a history of inappropriate laughter is present. Patients with ALS, a degenerative disease of upper and lower motor neurons characterized by muscle weakness and fasciculations, may also manifest episodes of inappropriate laughter. Dysarthria and dysphagia due to upper motor neuron disease is known as the pseudobulbar effect, and emotional lability with laughing and crying is a characteristic manifestation. Pseudobulbar palsy may also occur with advanced multiple sclerosis or bilateral strokes. Diagnosis of ALS is mainly clinically based on widespread motor neuron signs, although electromyography is an important diagnostic tool. Riluzole, an oral glutamate antagonist, may benefit some patients with ALS, but the disease is ultimately fatal.

ADDITIONAL READING

1. **Golbe LI, Davis PH, Schoenberg BS, et al.** Prevalence and natural history of progressive supranuclear palsy. Neurology 1988;38:1031.
2. **Rowland LP.** Diagnosis of amyotrophic lateral sclerosis. J Neurol Sci 1998;160(suppl 1):S6.

23

Loss of Taste for Cigarettes

Significance: The sudden taste aversion for smoking in a smoker is a characteristic symptom of acute viral hepatitis.

ETIOLOGY

Acute viral hepatitis
  Hepatitis A
  Hepatitis B
  Hepatitis C
  Delta hepatitis
  Hepatitis E

DISCUSSION

A peculiar, but characteristic, symptom of acute viral hepatitis is a sudden distaste for cigarettes in a regular smoker. Acute viral hepatitis refers to an acute illness characterized by diffuse inflammation of the liver parenchyma due to several hepatotrophic viruses, usually hepatitis A or

B. Acquisition of hepatitis A is usually fecal-oral and via the parenteral or sexual route for hepatitis B. After an incubation period of 1 to 6 weeks, an acute illness characterized by malaise, fever, arthralgias, abdominal pain, dark urine, and jaundice ensues. Some patients may be so severely ill that they are unable to function. A characteristic symptom, however, of acute viral hepatitis is the sudden distaste for cigarettes (in a smoker), alcohol, and protein-containing foods, a phenomenon known as dysgeusia. The precise etiology of this symptom is unclear. Patients with symptoms of acute viral hepatitis should have liver transaminases and bilirubin assessed and, if abnormal, should undergo serologic testing for hepatitis A and B viruses, and, if suspected, hepatitis C as well. Treatment of acute hepatitis is generally supportive.

ADDITIONAL READING

1. **Henkin RI, Smith RF.** Hyposmia in acute viral hepatitis. Lancet 1971;1:823.
2. **Koff RS.** Hepatitis A. Lancet 1998;351:1643.

Numbness of the Lip and Chin

Significance: Unilateral numbness of the chin and lip, also known as mental neuropathy or numb chin syndrome, may be a harbinger of metastatic cancer and results from compression of the inferior alveolar or mental nerve.

ETIOLOGY

Metastatic cancer
  Breast
  Lung
  Lymphoma
  Renal cell carcinoma
  Gastrointestinal tract
Acute leukemia
Trauma
Multiple sclerosis
Dental infections
Vasculitis
Mandibular osteomyelitis
Amyloidosis

DISCUSSION

The seemingly trivial symptom of lip, chin, or gingival numbness may signal the presence of life-threatening disease, notably, metastatic cancer. Numb chin syndrome, or mental neuropathy, refers to unilateral numbness or anesthesia of the areas innervated by the mental nerve, a sensory branch of the inferior alveolar nerve. The inferior alveolar nerve is a branch of the third division (V3) of the trigeminal nerve, a mixed motor and sensory cranial nerve. After passing through the mandible, the inferior alveolar nerve continues as the mental nerve as it exits the mental foramen. The mental nerve supplies sensory innervation to the skin of the chin, the lip, and the gingiva around the mandibular incisors. Typically, a metastatic lesion of the mandible compresses the inferior alveolar or mental nerve. However, some cases result from leukemic cell infiltration of the nerve sheath or compression by non-malignant processes. Symptoms of chin, lip, or gingival numbness may be the first manifestation of cancer or may occur in patients with known disease. Physical examination reveals decreased sensation of the chin, lip, and gingiva. Diagnosis of numb chin syndrome relies on recognizing the clinical significance of nontraumatic chin numbness followed by imaging studies. A panoramic radiograph of the mandible often reveals a lytic lesion, although nuclear bone scanning or magnetic resonance imaging may be useful in some cases. Evidence of metastatic disease is usually apparent in patients with cancer-associated numb chin syndrome. Treatment depends on the underlying etiology of numb chin syndrome, but in the case of malignancy, treatment is usually palliative and may consist of chemotherapy or radiation.

ADDITIONAL READING

1. **Marinella MA.** Metastatic large cell lung cancer presenting with numb chin syndrome. Respir Med 1997;91:235.
2. **Marinella MA.** Numb chin syndrome: a subtle clue to possible serious illness. Hosp Physician 2000;36:54.

Pain After Drinking Alcohol

Significance: Pain after consuming alcohol is a peculiar symptom that uncommonly occurs in patients with malignancy, usually Hodgkin's lymphoma.

ETIOLOGY

Hodgkin's lymphoma
Non-Hodgkin's lymphoma
Cervical cancer
Head and neck cancer
Breast cancer
Endometrial cancer
Bladder cancer

DISCUSSION

Pain after consuming alcohol is a peculiar, and often unrecognized, symptom of underlying malignancy, most commonly Hodgkin's lymphoma. Pain typically occurs in affected lymph node areas of the neck, chest, and abdomen. Patients with cancer of the bladder or cervix occasionally experience pelvic pain. Pain usually occurs within minutes of alcohol consumption, but may be delayed for several hours. The amount of alcohol necessary to produce pain in affected patients may be as little as one or two sips. Alcohol-induced pain often precedes diagnosis of malignancy, sometimes by months or years. The pain has been described by some patients as very severe or unlike any type of pain previously experienced. Alcohol-induced pain usually remits after successful therapy for the underlying neoplasm. The incidence of this unusual symptom is unknown, although some studies report an incidence of approximately 20% in patients with Hodgkin's disease. As such, clinicians should perform a thorough physical examination in any patient with pain after alcohol consumption and consider additional imaging studies to exclude underlying malignancy. Treatment of this peculiar symptom includes avoidance of alcoholic beverages and therapy directed at the primary malignancy.

ADDITIONAL READING

1. **Brewin TB.** Alcohol intolerance in neoplastic disease. Br Med J 1966;2:437.

Pain in the First Metatarsophalangeal Joint

Significance: Acute, severe pain in the first metatarsophalangeal joint, known as podagra, is classically associated with gouty arthritis, but can uncommonly occur with other disorders.

ETIOLOGY

Gout
Pseudogout
Rheumatoid arthritis
Osteoarthritis
Sarcoidosis
Psoriatic arthritis
Reiter's syndrome
Inflammatory bowel disease
Septic arthritis
Hemochromatosis

DISCUSSION

Podagra, a Greek term for "pain in the foot," refers to severe pain involving the first metatarsophalangeal joint and is classically associated with acute gouty arthropathy. Gout is the most common etiology of podagra and usually results from renal underexcretion of uric acid, although overproduction of urate may occur in the setting of hematologic malignancy or congenital enzyme deficiencies. The pain of podagra due to acute gout is very severe and is exacerbated by the slightest touch, such as that of a bed sheet. The metatarsophalangeal joint is usually warm, erythematous, and very tender to palpation. Arthrocentesis reveals needle-shaped birefringent crystals within the cytoplasm of neutrophils. Pseudogout, arthropathy due to deposition of calcium pyrophosphate dihydrate, is clinically similar to gout and may produce podagra on occasion. In addition, there are several other conditions that may result in podagra. However, acute gouty arthritis is the most common etiology of podagra, and patients with this symptom should be evaluated and treated accordingly. In patients with gout, agents such as indomethacin, colchicine, and corticosteroids may be effective.

ADDITIONAL READING

1. **Bomalaski JS, Schumacher HR.** Podagra is more than gout. Bull Rheum Dis 1984;34:1.
2. **George TM, Mandell BF.** Individualizing the treatment of gout. Cleve Clin J Med 1996;63:150.

27

Pain in the Tongue During Chewing

Significance: Tongue pain that occurs during chewing, masticatory claudication, results from poor blood flow through the lingual artery and is usually a complication of giant cell arteritis.

ETIOLOGY

Giant cell arteritis
Atherosclerosis
Embolism to the lingual artery

DISCUSSION

Lingual, or masticatory, claudication is a peculiar symptom that is most commonly associated with giant cell arteritis, a large vessel granulomatous arteritis occurring in patients over 50 years of age. Giant cell arteritis has a predilection for the extracranial arteries of the skull, but may also involve branches of the aorta, internal carotid, and vertebral arteries. Headache and visual symptoms are the most common symptoms associated with giant cell arteritis, but lingual claudication has been reported to occur in up to 25% of patients. Patients typically note tongue pain while chewing food that resolves when chewing is discontinued. Patients may also note pallor of their tongue during episodes of pain. Overt lingual necrosis has been reported as a complication of giant cell arteritis and is due to vasculitic occlusion of the lingual artery, which leads to ischemic necrosis of lingual tissue. Tongue pain can be elicited by having the patient repetitively protrude his or her tongue. Patients with lingual claudication should have measurement of the erythrocyte sedimentation rate, which is almost always elevated in patients with giant cell arteritis. Temporal artery biopsy is the gold standard for diagnosis and reveals granulomatous infiltration and disruption of the internal elastic lamina. Arteriography of the carotid artery may reveal partial or complete occlusion of the lingual artery in patients with lingual artery involvement. Patients with giant cell arteritis must be treated expediently with corticosteroids to decrease the chances of visual loss.

ADDITIONAL READING

1. **Ginzburg E, Evans WE, Smith W.** Lingual infarction: a review of the literature. Ann Vasc Surg 1992;6:450.
2. **Sofferman RA.** Lingual infarction in cranial arteritis. JAMA 1980;243:2422.

Pain in Both Thighs Accompanied by Fever

Significance: Bilateral anterior thigh pain in a febrile patient has been noted to be a useful predictor of bacteremia.

ETIOLOGY

Bacteremia of various causes
  Urosepsis
  Pneumonia
  Endocarditis

DISCUSSION

Generalized myalgias are not unusual in patients with systemic infections and may be quite disabling. Myalgias likely result from various inflammatory mediators released from leukocytes in the setting of the systemic inflammatory response syndrome. A helpful historical clue to the presence of underlying bacteremia in a febrile patient is bilateral anterior thigh pain. The etiology of localized thigh myalgias in the presence of bacteremia may be due to localized, sterile inflammation or ischemia due to inflammation of small muscular arterioles. Myalgias localized to the trapezius muscles have also been reported with bacteremia due to endocarditis. Evaluation of a febrile patient with bilateral thigh pain should include a meticulous physical examination, as well as blood cultures. In a patient with bilateral thigh pain and evidence of bacteremia or sepsis, antibiotic therapy should be instituted based on the most likely source of systemic infection.

ADDITIONAL READING

1. **Louria DB, Sen P, Kapila KR, *et al*.** Anterior thigh pain or tenderness: a diagnostically useful manifestation of bacteremia. Arch Intern Med 1985;145:657.
2. **Marinella MA.** Group B streptococcal endocarditis presenting with bilateral trapezius myalgias. Int J Cardiol 1997;58:279.

Pain in the Legs While Walking Downhill

Significance: Exertional bilateral lower extremity pain that is relieved by walking uphill is suggestive of neurogenic claudication due to spinal stenosis.

ETIOLOGY

Idiopathic
Congenital
Degenerative disease
Osteoarthritis
Hypertrophy of ligamentum flavum
Spondylolisthesis
Spondylosis
Scoliosis
Rheumatoid arthritis
Ankylosing spondylitis
Metabolic disease
Paget's disease
Cushing's disease
Acromegaly
Pseudogout

DISCUSSION

Neurogenic claudication refers to lower extremity pain, and occasionally paresthesias, that results from a reduction in the diameter of the spinal canal. The spinal canal may be congenitally narrowed or may be narrowed by conditions that result in increased bony or ligamentous hypertrophy. Encroachment of bone, ligament, or disc on the contents of the neural structures within the spinal canal results in the characteristic symptomatology. Spinal stenosis is more common in men and usually presents in patients over 50 years of age. Back pain is common. However, the characteristic symptom of spinal stenosis is intermittent neurogenic claudication, which results in bilateral lower extremity pain and paresthesias that occur during standing and walking. Sitting promptly relieves the discomfort. Postures that result in extension of the lumbar spine, such as walking downhill or lying prone, exacerbate symptoms due to further narrowing of the spinal canal. However, postures that tend to flex the lumbar spine, such as walking uphill, classically relieve the symptoms and serve as a valuable historical clue to help differentiate neurogenic from vascular claudication. Diagnosis of spinal stenosis is suggested by a characteristic history, supplemented by a thorough neurologic and vascular examination and by imaging of the spinal canal with computed tomography or magnetic resonance imaging. Many patients with progressive or severe spinal stenosis require surgical decompression.

ADDITIONAL READING

1. **Alvarez JA, Hardy RH.** Lumbar spine stenosis: a common cause of back and leg pain. Am Fam Physician 1998;57:1825.
2. **Circillo SF, Weinstein PR.** Lumbar spinal stenosis. West J Med 1993;158:171.

Pain in the Spine in the Middle of the Night

Significance: Nocturnal back pain that is severe enough to awaken a patient is often associated with significant underlying pathology, notably malignancy.

ETIOLOGY

Malignancy
  Metastatic carcinoma (e.g., breast, lung, kidney, prostate, thyroid)
  Multiple myeloma
  Lymphoma
Vertebral osteomyelitis
Cauda equina tumor
Vertebral compression fracture

DISCUSSION

Back pain that awakens the patient at night is a worrisome symptom for significant underlying disease. Lumbar pain has a variety of etiologies, most of which are mechanical and due to lumbar muscle strain. Benign causes of back pain are usually acute in onset, relieved by rest, and resolve with conservative therapy. More sinister etiologies of back pain such as malignancy or infection tend to occur in patients over 50 years of age. In addition, other historical factors such as smoking, weight loss, and a prior history of cancer should alert the clinician to the potential of serious pathology, notably malignancy. Most cases of malignant back pain are due to metastases to the vertebral body but can also involve the epidural space, spinal cord, and other surrounding structures. The complaint of back pain in the middle of the night is an alarming symptom that is often associated with malignant or other serious inflammatory diseases. Nocturnal back pain may awaken the patient from sleep or prevent the patient from achieving a deep, restful sleep. The patient typically describes the pain as constant, dull, and unrelieved by rest. Characteristically, the pain is worsened in the supine position and is not relieved by lying motionless. Patients with nocturnal back pain should undergo a thorough history and physical examination, focusing on clues of metastatic cancer or systemic infection. In fact, approximately 90% of patients with malignant spine disease note a history of nocturnal back pain. Lumbar radiographs may reveal destructive vertebral lesions. However, magnetic resonance imaging should be performed for definitive diagnosis and to exclude spinal cord compression. Patients with malignancy-induced nocturnal back pain require therapy directed at the particular tumor type, and patients with osteomyelitis require long-term antibiotic therapy and occasionally surgery.

ADDITIONAL READING

1. **Deyo RA, Diehl AK.** Cancer as a cause of back pain. Frequency, clinical presentation, and diagnostic strategies. J Gen Intern Med 1988;3:230.
2. **Mazanec DJ.** Evaluating back pain in older patients. Cleve Clin J Med 1999;66:89.

31

Pain in a Leg During a Sneeze

Significance: Pain in the leg during a sneeze, especially over the distribution of the venous system, is an unusual symptom of venous thrombosis.

ETIOLOGY

Deep venous thrombosis
Superficial thrombophlebitis

DISCUSSION

Pain involving the anatomic distribution of the lower extremity venous circulation that occurs during a sneeze (Louvel's sign) is suggestive of acute venous thrombosis. Deep venous thrombosis is a common clinical occurrence and results from an interplay of Virchow's triad: endothelial damage, venous stasis, and hypercoagulability. There are many etiologies of venous thrombosis, including immobility, surgery, trauma, and malignancy, as well as inherited and acquired thrombophilic states. Superficial thrombophlebitis involves the superficial venous system (e.g., the saphenous vein and tributaries) and does not typically result in the morbidity and mortality associated with deep venous thrombosis. Symptoms of deep vein thrombosis are nonspecific and include extremity swelling, redness, warmth, and pain. Low-grade fever may occur as well. An unusual, but historically helpful, symptom is the presence of pain along the course of the thrombosed vein when the patient sneezes or coughs. The pain may disappear when the examiner digitally compresses the vein proximal to the thrombosis. The etiology of the pain may be due to changes in venous pressure generated by a sneeze or cough that are transmitted to the occluded vein. Patients suspected of having an acute venous thrombosis should undergo duplex ultrasonography. Treatment of deep venous thrombosis consists of immediate therapy with unfractionated heparin or low-molecular-weight heparin followed by warfarin therapy.

ADDITIONAL READING

1. **Davies IJT.** Clinical signs of deep-vein thrombosis. Lancet 1972;1:321.
2. **DeGowin RL, Brown DD.** Thorax: respiratory, cardiovascular, and lymphatic systems. In: DeGowin's Diagnostic examination. 7th ed. New York: McGraw-Hill, 2000:247–293.

32

Pain and Swelling of the Ears on a Recurrent Basis

Significance: Recurrent, painful swelling of the cartilaginous portion of the external ears, sparing the fleshy lobule, is a characteristic symptom of relapsing polychondritis.

ETIOLOGY

Relapsing polychondritis

DISCUSSION

The symptom of recurrent, painful swelling and redness of the cartilaginous portion of both ears is the most common manifestation of relapsing polychondritis, an inflammatory disease of unclear etiology that results in inflammation of cartilage of the ears, respiratory system, nose, and joints. Pathologically, cartilage of involved tissues is infiltrated with inflammatory cells with loss of matrix staining and fibrosis. The etiology of relapsing polychondritis is unknown, but immunologic factors likely play a substantial role. Involvement of the trachea and larynx resulting in stenosis and airway compromise are the most feared consequences of relapsing polychondritis and may lead to life-threatening airway obstruction. Although relapsing polychondritis not infrequently involves the joints, heart, skin, and genitalia, the cartilaginous portion of the external ear is the most common anatomic site initially involved. Episodic inflammation of the cartilaginous portion of the external ears is responsible for the classic symptoms of relapsing polychondritis. The acute onset of pain, redness, and tender swelling of the external ear, sparing the cartilage-free lobule, is the most helpful historical clue in the diagnosis of relapsing polychondritis. Repeated episodes of inflammation may result in cartilage loss leading to a deformed "cauliflower ear." Diagnosis of relapsing polychondritis is mainly clinical, based on characteristic cartilaginous tissue inflammation and destruction. Biopsy of involved sites may be useful in equivocal cases. Antiinflammatory agents may provide acute relief from ear inflammation, although some patients require corticosteroids or immunosuppressive agents administered under direction of a rheumatologist.

ADDITIONAL READING

1. **McAdam LP, O'Hanlan MA, Bluestone R, et al.** Relapsing polychondritis. Medicine 1976;55:193.
2. **Sarodia BD, Dasgupta A, Mehta AC.** Management of airway manifestations of relapsing polychondritis. Chest 1999;116: 1669.

33

Pain over the Cheek That Is Brief and Lancinating

Significance: Severe, lancinating pain that episodically occurs over one-half of the face, often after trivial stimulation, is characteristic of trigeminal neuralgia (tic douloureux).

ETIOLOGY

Trigeminal neuralgia
  Idiopathic
  Multiple sclerosis
  Vascular abnormality in the posterior fossa
  Tumor of posterior fossa
  Herpes zoster

DISCUSSION

The brief, intense unilateral facial pain characteristic of trigeminal neuralgia is often a vexing problem for afflicted patients. Trigeminal neuralgia is usually idiopathic. However, patients with multiple sclerosis or abnormalities within the posterior fossa may also develop symptoms. For instance, a multiple sclerosis plaque, tumor, or blood vessel may irritate the root of the trigeminal nerve within the brain stem. Most cases of trigeminal neuralgia occur in middle-aged or older patients. Identifying the classic symptom of severe, lancinating paroxysms of unilateral facial pain, often following minimal stimulation to the face, is essential to the diagnosis. The pain usually involves the lips, gums, cheek, and chin. Chewing, shaving, or lightly touching the skin in the area of the 2nd and 3rd divisions of the trigeminal nerve frequently precipitates pain, and patients often go to great lengths to avoid any stimulation whatsoever. Characteristically, trigeminal neuralgia is diagnosed by history, and physical examination reveals no abnormalities. If the history or physical examination suggests an underlying etiology such as multiple sclerosis, magnetic resonance imaging of the brain should be performed. However, the majority of cases are idiopathic and diagnosis is purely clinical. Treatment options include carbamazepine or other anticonvulsants. Some patients may be candidates for surgical correction.

ADDITIONAL READING

1. **Dalessio DJ.** Relief of cluster headache and cranial neuralgias. Postgrad Med 2001;109:69.
2. **Dalessio DJ.** Trigeminal neuralgia: a practical approach to treatment. Drugs 1982;24:248.

34

Persistent, Painful Erection

Significance: A persistent, painful erection, a condition known as priapism, results from increased blood volume within the penile shaft and may complicate underlying disorders such as sickle cell anemia.

ETIOLOGY

Sickle cell anemia
Drugs
   Trazadone
   Chlorpromazine
   Vancomycin
Intracavernosal papaverine/phentolamine
Metastatic tumor
   Transitional cell carcinoma
   Prostate cancer
   Gastrointestinal cancer
Leukemia
Thrombosis
Traumatic arterial-cavernosal fistula
Fabry's disease
Idiopathic

DISCUSSION

Priapism is the presence of a persistent, painful erection occurring in the absence of sexual stimulation. Normal penile erection is mediated by relaxation and contraction of smooth muscle cells present within the cavernosal sinuses and arterioles. Priapism may result from sluggish venous outflow from the cavernosal sinusoids or from increased arterial inflow into the cavernosal sinusoids. Trauma to the internal pudendal artery or its branches may result in an arterial-to-cavernosal shunt leading to massive arterial inflow that overwhelms venous outflow. Sickle cell disease may cause priapism due to small vessel occlusion by sickled erythrocytes. A thorough drug history should be obtained, as well as a general physical and genitourinary examination. Prolonged priapism may lead to permanent penile fibrosis from local ischemia and acidosis. A sickle cell screen or hemoglobin electrophoresis should be obtained in any black man with priapism if no prior history of sickle cell disease is present. Referral to a urologist is indicated for further evaluation and treatment that depends on the underlying etiology.

ADDITIONAL READING

1. **Harmon WJ, Nehra A**. Priapism: diagnosis and management. Mayo Clin Proc 1997;72:350.
2. **Powars DR, Johnson CS**. Priapism. Hematol Oncol Clin North Am 1996;10:1363.

35

Pruritus After
a Warm Bath

Significance: Aquagenic pruritus, pruritus that occurs after exposure to water, may be the initial manifestation of a hematologic disorder, typically polycythemia vera.

ETIOLOGY

Polycythemia vera
Myelodysplastic syndrome
Hypereosinophilic syndromes

DISCUSSION

Aquagenic pruritus is an unusual symptom that consists of itching and occasionally tingling of the skin after exposure to warm water, which classically occurs in association with polycythemia vera. Other hematologic conditions, however, have rarely been associated with this symptom. Many patients first report symptom onset after taking a warm shower or bath. In fact, some patients may not be able to tolerate bathing due to severe pruritus. There is no clear relationship between the degree of pruritus and the hematocrit since some patients with polycythemia vera may have aquagenic pruritus with a normal hematocrit. The etiology of pruritus is unclear, but may relate to increased circulating histamine levels, which have been demonstrated to occur with water exposure in patients with polycythemia vera. Increased levels of prostaglandins and platelet-derived inflammatory mediators (e.g., sero-tonin) may also play a role. Evaluation of patients with aquagenic pruritus should include a complete blood count periodically since symptoms in some patients may precede diagnosis of polycythemia vera. Treatment of aquagenic pruritus may be difficult, but some patients respond to hydroxyurea, aspirin, and antihistamines. Patients with aquagenic pruritus due to polycythemia vera often require phlebotomy.

ADDITIONAL READING

1. **Archer CB, Camp RDR, Greaves MW.** Polycythemia vera can present with aquagenic pruritus. Lancet 1988;1:1451.
2. **McGrath JA, Greaves MW, Warin AP.** Aquagenic pruritus and myelodysplastic syndrome. Am J Hematol 1991;37:63.

Pruritus of the Nostrils, Severe and Persistent

Significance: Severe pruritus of the nostrils, known as Wartenberg's symptom, is an uncommon, but characteristic, symptom of a brain neoplasm.

ETIOLOGY

Astrocytoma
Glioblastoma
Oligodendroglioma
Medulloblastoma
Metastatic tumors

DISCUSSION

Intense nasal pruritus, also known as Wartenberg's symptom, has been noted to be pathognomonic of an underlying brain neoplasm, usually a primary brain tumor. A study by Andreev *et al.* noted intense bilateral nostril pruritus in six of 77 patients with brain neoplasms. The pathogenesis is unclear, but all of these patients had advanced tumors with infiltration of the base of the fourth ventricle. Most patients experience severe, persistent pruritus that leads to intense scratching that often occurs during sleep. Patients are often consumed with scratching their nostrils, often to the point of mucosal irritation. Clinicians should consider brain imaging with either computed tomography or magnetic resonance imaging in patients with severe, persistent nostril pruritus. Treatment involves therapy directed at the primary tumor, which may include surgical resection, chemotherapy, or radiation therapy.

ADDITIONAL READING

1. **Andreev VC, Petkov I**. Skin manifestations associated with tumors of the brain. Br J Dermatol 1975;92:675.

Stools That Are Silver-Colored

Significance: Stool that appears silver or the color of aluminum paint is an unusual, but characteristic, symptom of a carcinoma of the ampulla of Vater.

ETIOLOGY

Carcinoma of the ampulla of Vater
Jaundice of pregnancy and oral iron therapy

DISCUSSION

Stool that appears silver or the color of aluminum paint (Thomas's sign) is a rare, but specific, finding for carcinoma of the ampulla of Vater. First described by A. M. Thomas, a British pathologist, silver stool has been reported in several patients with malignant tumors of the ampulla of Vater. The silver color results from the mixture of acholic (white) stools from biliary obstruction and blood that exudes from the tumor. Silver stool has also been reported to occur in a patient with jaundice of pregnancy who ingested iron tablets. Although a rare phenomenon, any patient who relays the history of silver-colored stool should be evaluated for hyperbilirubinemia and undergo imaging of the biliary system to exclude ampullary carcinoma. Optimal treatment of ampullary carcinoma is surgical resection if no evidence of metastatic disease is present. Otherwise, palliative surgical bypass procedures may be necessary in the case of intestinal obstruction.

ADDITIONAL READING

1. **Ogilvie H**. Thomas's sign, or silver stool in cancer of the ampulla of Vater. Br Med J 1955;1:208.
2. **Ong YYT, Pintauro WM**. Silver stools. JAMA 1979;242:2433.

38

Sweating and Flushing of the Cheek While Chewing

Significance: Sweating that occurs over the cheek area during food ingestion, or gustatory sweating, is known as Frey syndrome and typically follows surgery to the parotid gland.

ETIOLOGY

Parotidectomy
Radical neck dissection
Submaxillary gland surgery
Subcondylar fracture
Parotid gland trauma
Herpes zoster
Cisplatinum chemotherapy

DISCUSSION

Gustatory sweating is a characteristic symptom of Frey syndrome, a common complication of parotid gland surgery.

First described by Lucie Frey in 1923, Frey syndrome is probably most well known in the otolaryngology literature given the quite frequent association with head and neck surgeries, typically parotidectomy. However, other etiologies of this syndrome have been described. Normally, postganglionic sympathetic fibers innervate the sweat glands, and postganglionic parasympathetic fibers innervate the parotid gland. After surgical or traumatic damage to the parotid nerve fibers, aberrant regrowth of postganglionic parasympathetic cholinergic fibers to the sweat gland occurs. As a result, stimulation of these aberrant fibers with eating and mastication leads to a secremotor response resulting in sweating and vasodilation. The typical symptoms of Frey syndrome are mastication-related sweating and flushing of the skin anterior to the ear and angle of the mandible in the area of the parotid gland. Patients may also note nonspecific discomfort as well. Diagnosis of Frey syndrome is based on the typical history. However, diagnosis can be confirmed with the Minor test in which an iodine-starch solution is painted over the cheek area. The sweat imparts a blue color to the mixture. Treatment of Frey syndrome is difficult, although topical anticholinergic agents such as glycopyrrolate may benefit some patients.

ADDITIONAL READING

1. **Bonanno PC, Casson PR.** Frey's syndrome: a preventable phenomenon. Plast Reconstr Surg 1992;89:452.
2. **Dulguerov P, Quinodoz D, Cosendai G,** *et al*. Prevention of Frey syndrome during parotidectomy. Arch Otolaryngol Head Neck Surg 1999;125:833.

Syncope While Shaving

Significance: Syncope that occurs during activity that places pressure on the carotid artery, such as shaving, is very suggestive of carotid sinus hypersensitivity.

ETIOLOGY

Carotid sinus hypersensitivity
Atherosclerosis
Extrinsic tumor compression
Carotid body tumor
Cervical adenopathy
Prior neck radiation

DISCUSSION

Carotid sinus hypersensitivity is a form of episodic syncope precipitated by pressure on baroreceptors of the internal carotid artery. The carotid baroreceptors are located in the tunica adventitia cephalad to the carotid bifurcation in the neck. The carotid sinus baroreceptors are sensitive to stretch and pressure and send impulses via the nerve of Hering, a branch of the glossopharyngeal nerve, to the brain stem. Efferent impulses travel via the vagus nerves and sympathetic chain to the sinoatrial and atrioventricular nodes, as well as the peripheral vasculature. Stimulation of the carotid sinus typically results in a physiologic decrease in the heart rate, which is usually well tolerated. Patients with hypersensitivity of the carotid sinus, however, have a pathologic response that includes significant bradycardia or asystole (the cardioinhibitory response), significant hypotension (the vasodepressor response), or a mixed response. Patients with carotid sinus hypersensitivity may note dizziness, lightheadedness, and overt syncope with any maneuver that exerts pressure on the carotid sinus. Well-known precipitants of symptoms include a tight shirt collar, shaving over the neck, and vigorously turning the head to one side. Physical examination typically reveals bradycardia, hypotension, or both in response to massage of the carotid body. Care must be taken to avoid massage if significant carotid stenosis is present to avoid cerebral hypoperfusion and subsequent stroke. Patients with carotid sinus hypersensitivity often require implantation of a permanent pacemaker.

ADDITIONAL READING

1. **McIntosh SJ, Lawson J, Kenny RA.** Clinical characteristics of vasodepressor, cardioinhibitory, and mixed carotid sinus syndrome in the elderly. Am J Med 1993;95:203.
2. **Strasberg B, Sagie A, Erdman S, et al.** Carotid sinus hypersensitivity and the carotid sinus syndrome. Prog Cardiovasc Dis 1989;31:379.

Urine That Is Foamy

Significance: Urine that has a foamy appearance on voiding into the toilet or a specimen jar is characteristic of nephrotic syndrome.

ETIOLOGY

Nephrotic syndrome
  Diabetic nephropathy
  Minimal change disease
  Amyloidosis
  Intravenous drug use
  Paraneoplastic syndromes (e.g., Hodgkin's disease)
  Drugs (e.g., NSAIDs, gold, penicillamine, captopril)
  Systemic lupus erythematosus
  Systemic vasculitis
  Human immunodeficiency virus infection

DISCUSSION

Urine that has a foamy appearance on voiding into a toilet or a specimen container is considered a classic symptom of nephrotic syndrome. Nephrotic syndrome refers to the syndrome consisting of pathologic urine protein loss (>3.5 g over a 24-hour period), edema, hypoproteinemia, hyperlipidemia, and lipiduria. There are many etiologies of nephrotic syndrome as noted above, but diabetes mellitus is one of the most frequent causes in adults. Glomerular damage results in a breakdown of the size-selective and charge-selective barriers for protein conservation, thereby resulting in proteinuria. Albumin is the chief serum protein lost in the urine, although other proteins may be lost as well (e.g., antithrombin III loss can lead to venous thrombosis). Albuminuria leads to protein malnutrition, as well as the hallmark physical sign of nephrotic syndrome, severe generalized edema. The urine of patients with nephrotic syndrome is rich in albumin and other proteins and, when voided, characteristically "foams" in the container or toilet. This foaming is due to the increased protein content and may be an initial curious complaint noted by the patient. Evaluation of patients with suspected nephrotic syndrome should include a 24-hour quantitative urine protein determination, as well as a serum albumin level. Once nephrotic syndrome is confirmed, a careful search for the underlying etiology should ensue. Primary therapy of nephrotic syndrome depends on the etiology, but many patients require loop diuretics for volume overload.

ADDITIONAL READING

1. **Orth SR, Ritz E.** The nephrotic syndrome. N Engl J Med 1998;338;1202.
2. **Schnaper HW, Robson AM.** Nephrotic syndrome: minimal change disease, focal glomerulosclerosis, and related disorders. In: Diseases of the kidney. 6th ed. Boston: Little, Brown and Company, 1998:1725–1780.

Urine That Is Brown upon First Morning Void

Significance: A reddish-brown urine color recurrently present upon the first morning void is suggestive of the intravascular hemolysis complicating paroxysmal nocturnal hemoglobinuria (PNH).

ETIOLOGY

Paroxysmal nocturnal hemoglobinuria

DISCUSSION

Nocturnal episodes of intravascular hemolysis may impart a reddish-brown color to the urine that is notably visible upon the first morning void. PNH is an acquired clonal hematopoietic stem cell disorder that results in episodic intravascular hemolysis. The red cell membrane in patients with PNH possesses an abnormal sensitivity to lysis by serum complement, which results in recurrent episodes of intravascular hemolysis, especially during times of stress such as infection. PNH classically causes nocturnal hemolysis since the respiratory acidosis that normally accompanies sleep leads to increased complement activity and subsequent hemolysis. Patients may note their first morning urine to be reddish brown, which results from glomerular hemoglobin loss that is not resorbed by the renal tubular cells. Patients suspected of having PNH should undergo a complete blood count since some cases can be associated with aplastic anemia. Evidence of intravascular hemolysis includes indirect hyperbilirubinemia, an elevated lactate dehydrogenase, and the presence of urine hemosiderin. Patients with a history of recurrent reddish-brown morning urine should undergo an acid hemolysis test (Hamm's test) in which blood is incubated with hydrochloric acid; a positive test is present if hemolysis occurs after 1 hour. Flow cytometric analysis of the peripheral blood is very sensitive and specific to confirm the diagnosis. Treatment of PNH often requires blood transfusion and folic acid supplementation. Bone marrow transplantation has been successful in some patients.

ADDITIONAL READING

1. **Hillmen P, Lewis SM, Bessler M, et al.** Natural history of paroxysmal nocturnal hemoglobinuria. N Engl J Med 1995;333: 1253.
2. **Rotoli B, Luzzatto L.** Paroxysmal nocturnal hemoglobinuria. Baillieres Clin Haematol 1989;2:113.

Urine That Smells Like Maple Syrup

Significance: The symptom of urine that smells like maple syrup is characteristic of maple syrup urine disease, an inborn error of metabolism resulting in elevated serum and urine levels of branched chain amino acids.

ETIOLOGY

Maple syrup urine disease (MSUD)
    Neonatal form
    Intermittent form (may present in adulthood)
    Thiamine-responsive MSUD

DISCUSSION

Urine that smells like maple syrup is a characteristic symptom of MSUD, an autosomal recessive inborn error of metabolism. MSUD results from deficiency of the mito-chondrial branched-chain alpha-ketoacid dehydrogenase complex that results in the accumulation of the branched-chain amino acids leucine, isoleucine, and valine. Elevated blood levels of these amino acids leads to increased urinary excretion, as well as to increased urine levels of sotolone, a compound also found in maple syrup. Patients with MSUD usually develop overt manifestations during the neonatal period such as seizures, coma, and severe metabolic acidosis. The accumulation of branched-chain amino acids often leads to irreversible neurologic damage. Occasional patients may manifest an intermittent form of MSUD that becomes symptomatic during adulthood complicating stressful periods such as surgery, trauma, or infection. The classic symptom of urine and sweat that smells like maple syrup may be relayed by the patient or caregiver. Intermittent ataxia and confusion may be present in the intermittent form of MSUD. Patients suspected of having MSUD should have plasma and urinary levels of leucine, isoleucine, and valine measured. Dietary intake of the branched-chain amino acids should be limited as soon as possible.

ADDITIONAL READING

1. **Asola MR.** A diver unconscious after gastroenteritis. Lancet 1995;346:1338.
2. **Podebrad F, Heil M, Reichert S, et al.** 4,5-dimethyl-3-hydroxy-2[5H]-furanone (sotolone)—the odor of maple syrup urine disease. J Inherit Metabol Dis 1999;22:107.

Urine or Sweat That Smells Like Sweaty Feet

Significance: The intermittent odor resembling sweaty feet affecting the urine or body fluids such as sweat is a characteristic symptom of isovaleric acidemia, which results from deficiency of isovaleryl CoA dehydrogenase.

ETIOLOGY

Isovaleric acidemia
  Acute neonatal form
  Chronic intermittent form

DISCUSSION

Urine or sweat odor that resembles sweaty feet is a characteristic symptom of the autosomal recessive metabolic disease of leucine metabolism known as isovaleric acidemia. Deficiency of the enzyme isovaleryl CoA dehydrogenase leads to elevated plasma levels of isovaleric acid, which results in ketoacidosis and progressive neurologic dysfunction and hematologic abnormalities such as neutropenia and thrombocytopenia. The acute form of isovaleric acidemia presents in the neonatal period. However, some patients are afflicted with a chronic intermittent form that may only become symptomatic during early adulthood following the stress of infection, trauma, or surgery. Acute acidotic episodes may also complicate overingestion of dietary protein. The classic symptom of isovaleric acidemia is the distinctive odor of the urine and sweat that resembles sweaty feet and is due to the increased isovaleric acid levels. Interestingly, patients with the chronic intermittent form of the disease may develop an aversion to protein-rich foods. Diagnosis of isovaleric acidemia may be delayed in adults due to the rarity of the disease. Measurement of isovaleric acid in the plasma is essential for diagnosis and should be performed if the characteristic sweaty feet odor is noted. Treatment includes dietary leucine restriction, although some patients may benefit from glycine or carnitine supplements.

ADDITIONAL READING

1. **Budd MA, Tanaka K, Holmes LB, *et al*.** Isovaleric acidemia—clinical features of a new genetic defect of leucine metabolism. N Engl J Med 1967;277:321.
2. **Sweetman L, Williams JC.** Branched chain organic acidurias. In: The metabolic and molecular basis of inherited disease. Scriver CR, Beaudet AL, Sly WS, Valle D, eds. 7th ed. New York: McGraw-Hill, Inc., 1995:1387–1422.

44

Urine That Turns Brown Accompanied by Flank Pain After Cold Exposure

Significance: The symptom of brownish colored urine and flank pain after exposure to cold ambient temperature is suggestive of the cold-induced hemolytic anemias paroxysmal cold hemoglobinuria (PCH) or cold-agglutinin disease.

ETIOLOGY

Paroxysmal cold hemoglobinuria
   Viral illness
   Syphilis
   Malignancy
Cold-agglutinin disease
   Mycoplasma infections
   Mononucleosis
   Malignancy
   Systemic lupus erythematosus

DISCUSSION

The symptom of brown urine that occurs after exposure to the cold is suggestive of the cold-induced hemolytic anemias PCH and cold-agglutinin disease. Paroxysmal cold hemoglobinuria is a rare etiology of autoimmune hemolytic anemia that historically complicated syphilitic infections, but now is usually associated with recent viral illnesses such as varicella, mumps, measles, and influenza. Hemolysis results from the presence of a cold-reacting IgG antibody directed at the erythrocyte P-antigen. This antibody preferentially binds to red cells at cold temperatures and subsequently binds complement on rewarming, which leads to hemolysis. The symptoms of PCH include the sudden onset of chills, malaise, and flank pain. The classic symptom, however, is brown urine, which results from hemoglobinuria. Diagnosis of PCH is based on history and supported by evidence of anemia, reticulocytosis, hemoglobinuria, and an elevated lactate dehydrogenase. The diagnosis of PCH can be confirmed with the Donath-Landsteiner test, which detects the presence of the cold hemolysin that attaches to red cells at 4°C and causes hemolysis when the specimen is heated to 37°C.

Cold-agglutinin disease occurs when a cold autoantibody (usually IgM) reacts with red cell surface antigens (usually the I-antigen) at cold temperatures. Recent mycoplasma infection and mononucleosis are frequent precipitants of cold-agglutinin disease. The red cell I-antigen is the typical target associated with mycoplasma infection and the i-antigen with mononucleosis. The symptoms and laboratory findings are similar to PCH, although rouleaux formation is common on the peripheral blood smear with cold-agglutinin disease. Measurement of serum cold-agglutinins confirms the diagnosis. Patients should avoid prolonged cold exposure. Specific therapy toward syphilis should be provided if infection is present, although this is a rare occurrence today.

ADDITIONAL READING

1. **Nicol SL, Harmening DM, Green R.** Hemolytic anemias: extra-corpuscular defects. In: Clinical hematology and fundamentals of hemostasis. Harmening DM, ed. 3rd ed. Philadelphia: F.A. Davis, 1997:221–243.
2. **Sharara AI, Hillsley RE, Wax TD, *et al*.** Paroxysmal cold hemo-globinuria associated with non-Hodgkin's lymphoma. South Med J 1994;87:397.

45

Urine with Gas Bubbles

Significance: Pneumaturia refers to the passage of gas in the urine and usually signifies a fistulous connection between the intestinal and urinary tracts.

ETIOLOGY

Colovesical fistula
    Diverticulitis
    Neoplasm
    Inflammatory bowel disease
    Surgical trauma
Urinary tract manipulation
Cystoscopy
Catheter insertion
Urinary tract infection
Emphysematous pyelonephritis
Emphysematous cystitis
Salpingoenteric fistula
Pelvic inflammatory disease

DISCUSSION

Pneumaturia is an unusual symptom referring to the passage of gas in the urine and is usually associated with a colovesical fistula due to complicated diverticulitis, although several other etiologies have been described as noted above. Patients may note gas bubbles within the urinary stream or have intermittent episodes of the passage of fetid-smelling gas. Dysuria and fecaluria may also be present if pneumaturia results from a colovesical fistula. Patients may report a history of fever and frequent urinary tract infections due to stool contamination of the normally sterile urinary tract. However, occasionally urinary tract infections due to gas-producing enteric bacteria may produce pneumaturia in the absence of any fistulous connection. In these instances, the gas has no odor, but contains varying amounts of carbon dioxide. Assessment of the patient with pneumaturia should include a complete physical examination with attention to the lower abdomen, urinalysis, urine culture, and imaging studies such as intravenous pyelography, cystoscopy, or barium enema to exclude a fistulous connection. Surgery is usually necessary in patients with pneumaturia due to a colovesical fistula. Antibiotics should be administered if a urinary tract infection is present.

ADDITIONAL READING

1. **Jain H, Greenblatt JM, Albornoz AM.** Emphysematous pyelonephritis: a rare case of pneumaturia. Lancet 2001;357:194.
2. **Synhaivsky A, Malek RS.** Isolated pneumaturia. Am J Med 1985;78:617.

46

Urine That Turns Black upon Standing

Significance: Urine that turns black upon standing is very suggestive of alkaptonuria, an autosomal recessive disorder of tyrosine metabolism.

ETIOLOGY

Alkaptonuria
Melanoma

DISCUSSION

Urine that turns black upon standing is very suggestive, if not pathognomonic, of the autosomal recessive disorder alkaptonuria. Alkaptonuria is a rare disorder of tyrosine metabolism characterized by deficiency of the enzyme homogentisic acid oxidase, which leads to the production of excessive amounts of homogentisic acid. Homogentisic acid polymerizes and deposits in connective tissues in such areas as the dermis, eyes, skeleton, and cardiac valves. This deposition of homogentisic acid is responsible for the characteristic findings, including black pigmentation of the skin and sclera, large joint arthropathy, and, occasionally, aortic valve stenosis. Characteristic symptoms of alkaptonuria include joint pain and dyspnea if aortic stenosis is severe. Homogentisic acid is excreted by the kidney. Freshly voided urine appears normal. However, upon standing, urine turns the characteristic black color that is virtually pathognomonic for alkaptonuria. Rarely, melanoma involving the genitourinary system can impart a black pigmentation to the urine that is usually present upon voiding. Diagnosis of alkaptonuria can be confirmed by adding Benedict's solution to fresh urine, which results in a black supernatant. Homogentisic acid levels are increased in the urine when tested with chromatography. There is no specific therapy for alkaptonuria, but patients with arthritis usually require analgesia and occasionally joint replacement. Rare patients may require aortic valve replacement.

ADDITIONAL READING

1. **Albers SE, Brozena SJ, Glass F, *et al.*** Alkaptonuria and ochronosis: case report and review. J Am Acad Dermatol 1992;27:609.
2. **Srsen S.** Alkaptonuria. Johns Hopkins Med J 1979;145:217.

47

Vertigo with Arm Exertion

Significance: Vertigo or other symptoms of vertebrobasilar ischemia that occur during vigorous upper extremity movements are suggestive of subclavian artery stenosis, also known as subclavian steal syndrome.

ETIOLOGY

Atherosclerosis
Takayasu's arteritis
Giant cell arteritis

DISCUSSION

Symptoms of vertebrobasilar insufficiency (e.g., vertigo, dysarthria, syncope, diplopia) that occur in the presence of a significant stenosis of the subclavian artery proximal to the origin of the ipsilateral vertebral artery constitute the subclavian steal syndrome. At rest, blood flow occurs normally across the stenosed artery. However, if the upper extremity is exercised, retrograde blood flow from the circle of Willis to the stenosed subclavian artery may lead to cerebrovascular ischemia. The term "subclavian steal" emanates from the concept that the stenosed subclavian artery "steals" the retrograde blood flow from the vertebral artery to increase extremity perfusion during exertion. Subclavian steal syndrome is rare and usually occurs in the setting of significant atherosclerotic disease. Rare cases may occur due to vasculitis of the large arteries. Diagnosis is suspected by the historical clue of vertebrobasilar ischemic symptoms during significant movement of the upper extremity. Stenosis of the subclavian artery leads to a lower blood pressure in the involved extremity, which also enhances the "steal" phenomenon from the higher-pressure proximal circulation. Symptoms of arm claudication may occur in some patients. Physical manifestations include a discrepancy in upper extremity blood pressure, a reduced or absent radial pulse, and a bruit over the supraclavicular fossa. Confirmation of the diagnosis can be obtained by Doppler ultrasound, magnetic resonance angiography, or conventional angiography. Treatment of subclavian steal may be difficult, but may include antithrombotic therapy with aspirin and cholesterol lowering drugs. Patients should avoid motions that produce symptoms, although some patients may require angioplasty or surgical bypass of the stenotic arterial lesion.

ADDITIONAL READING

1. **Gosselin C, Walker PM.** Subclavian steal syndrome: existence, clinical features, diagnosis and management. Semin Vasc Surg 1996;9:93.
2. **Miller-Fisher C.** A new vascular syndrome—"the subclavian steal." N Engl J Med 1962;265:1912.

48

Visual Loss That Occurs Suddenly—Like a Window Shade Pulled Down

Significance: Acute monocular vision loss, often likened to a shade being pulled over one's eye, is known as amaurosis fugax and usually occurs with transient retinal ischemia due to cholesterol plaque embolization from the carotid circulation.

ETIOLOGY

Atherosclerosis of the carotid artery
Atrial fibrillation
Ventricular thrombus
Valvular disease
Giant cell arteritis
Takayasu's arteritis
Migraine headache
Hypercoagulable disorders
Paraproteinemias
Prosthetic cardiac valves

DISCUSSION

Transient monocular visual loss, or amaurosis fugax, is typically a manifestation of a transient ischemic attack of the carotid circulation. If blood flow to the retina is decreased for only a few seconds, visual loss occurs. The arterial supply to the retina is derived from the internal carotid artery. Patients with atherosclerotic plaques involving the internal carotid artery are most at risk for amaurosis fugax, as well as other symptoms of cerebral ischemia. Patients with high-grade carotid stenosis (70% to 99%) of the carotid artery are at a higher risk for cerebral ischemia than patients with lesser degrees of stenosis. If a small plaque embolizes and lodges in the retinal arteriolar circulation, patients may describe sudden, transient visual loss often compared with a shade being pulled over the field of vision. The visual loss usually lasts only a few minutes if the plaque breaks up or passes distally. Examination of the fundus may reveal the cholesterol emboli (Hollenhorst plaque). Some cases of amaurosis fugax result from vasospasm, fibrin-platelet emboli, or cardiogenic emboli. Other less common causes are noted above, but include vasculitis or hypercoagulable disorders. Patients with amaurosis fugax should undergo imaging of the carotid arteries with duplex ultrasonography followed by angiography if a significant stenosis is present. Treatment of atherosclerotic amaurosis fugax consists of aspirin and lipid lowering agents, as well as control of diabetes and hypertension. Smoking cessation is mandatory in such patients. Patients with significant carotid stenosis may benefit from endarterectomy.

ADDITIONAL READING

1. **Bernard GA, Bennett G.** Vasospastic amaurosis fugax. Arch Ophthalmol 1999;117:1568.

49

Visual Changes with Yellow-Green Halos Seen Around Lights

Significance: The symptom of yellow-green halos surrounding objects is suggestive of digoxin toxicity.

ETIOLOGY

Digoxin toxicity
    Overdosage
    Volume depletion
    Drug interaction (e.g., verapamil, amiodarone, antibiotics)
    Hypokalemia
    Hypomagnesemia
    Hypercalcemia
    Renal failure

DISCUSSION

The complaint of yellow-green halos around various objects is a useful indicator of digoxin toxicity. Digitalis glycosides have been used for years in the treatment of cardiac failure and are derived from various plant species, including foxglove, oleander, and lily of the valley. Digoxin, the most commonly utilized glycoside, is still widely used in patients with atrial fibrillation and systolic heart failure. Digoxin binds to a receptor on the cardiac myocyte, inactivating the sodium-potassium ATPase pump. This inactivation leads to increased intracellular calcium concentrations, which are responsible for the inotropic effects. The digitalis glycosides, however, possess a narrow therapeutic-toxic margin, which not infrequently leads to toxic effects, especially in elderly individuals who often take several medications and have a lower creatinine clearance. Digoxin intoxication more commonly occurs accidentally, and the symptoms are nonspecific, including nausea, vomiting, weakness, headache, and disorientation. A helpful symptom for the clinician, however, is the presence of yellow-green halos appearing around objects and light sources. It has been stated that the renowned artist Vincent Van Gogh chronically ingested foxglove, which may have caused halos to appear around lights and influenced many of his paintings. If digoxin toxicity is suspected, the digoxin level, as well as creatinine and electrolytes, should be measured. The patient should also be observed for cardiac arrhythmias. Treatment of digoxin toxicity requires discontinuation of the drug, hydration, correction of electrolyte imbalance, and use of digoxin antibody fragments ("Digibind") in cases of severe, acute toxicity.

ADDITIONAL READING

1. **Bayer MJ.** Recognition and management of digitalis intoxication: implications for emergency medicine. Am J Emerg Med 1991;9:29.
2. **Piltz JR, Wertenbaker C, Lance SE, et al.** Digoxin toxicity: recognizing the varied visual presentations. J Clin Neuro Ophthalmol 1993;13:275.

50

Visual Loss During a Hot Shower

Significance: Decreased visual acuity that occurs in a warm environment such as a shower, Uthoff's phenomenon, is suggestive of multiple sclerosis.

ETIOLOGY

Multiple sclerosis

DISCUSSION

Decreased visual acuity that occurs with increased body temperature (Uthoff's phenomenon) is a well-described entity that may occur in patients with multiple sclerosis. Common precipitants of this phenomenon include a hot bath or shower, increased outdoor temperature, exercise, and fever. Subclinical demyelination of the optic nerve is present in most of these patients. In addition, nerve conduction decreases to a pathologic degree in demyelinated nerves. Changes in sodium and potassium flux around the myelin sheath in response to higher temperature have been proposed based on mammalian studies. Uthoff's phenomenon may occur in patients without prior clinical involvement of the optic nerve. Other symptoms of neurologic dysfunction such as paresthesia and dysarthria may also occur with increased body temperature. The hot bath test has been reported by some authors to be helpful in the diagnosis of multiple sclerosis. Visual abnormalities were described by Malhorta *et al.* in the majority of patients with established multiple sclerosis who were immersed in bath water of 43°C. Clinicians should consider cerebral imaging studies to assess for changes of multiple sclerosis in any patient who notes visual or other neurologic complaints when exposed to increased temperatures. Treatment of patients with multiple sclerosis is very complex and requires referral to an experienced neurologist.

ADDITIONAL READING

1. **Malhotra AS, Goren H.** The hot bath test in the diagnosis of multiple sclerosis. JAMA 1981;246:1113.
2. **Guthrie TC.** Visual and motor changes in patients with multiple sclerosis: a result of induced changes in environmental temperatures. Arch Neurol Psychiatry 1951;65:437.

Index